A STROKE OF
LIFE

B. FRANCES SPENCER

ISBN: 979-8-90252-054-2   (Paperback)
ISBN: 979-8-90252-053-5   (eBook)

Printed in the United States of America

Greetings to all.

This book is about my return from death. Yes, I said my return from the threshold of death.

First, I will introduce myself. I have been a nurse for thirty-two plus years. I have worked in every area of nursing except labour and delivery, and yet when I was having a stroke, I had no idea what I was experiencing. Maybe the signs were there, but I did not notice them. I was too busy working and taking care of my sister, who needed me more than ever. But I can tell you, it doesn't always happen the way the textbook says, and each person's case is different.

It was on a Friday, in October. After work I visited my sister; our visit lasted till about 9:00 p.m. I got home, bathed, and was talking to a friend from Nigeria. He said that I told him I was going to New York in the morning. At that point, I started to be confused, because I had no plans of travelling to New York that morning or anytime soon.

I found myself walking around my bedroom, trying to contact my daughter, who lived on the third floor. I was in the basement at the time. I thought about taking the stairs, but I had three flights of eight steps each. Something told me not to do it, because my daughter could be listening to music or sleeping, and she would not hear me. I also thought about stopping on the first floor, but the tenant's daughter there could be sleeping, so I decided against it. I started to open the door that leads to the outside, but something held me back.

You see, I have a sunken driveway, if I fall the tenant may drive over me not knowing I was there, which would be a disaster. All this time I was in my confused state making decisions that could save my life because my ancestors were talking to me. I tried to open the door, it was difficult but eventually I turned the lock. I didn't have the strength to turn the knob, so I decided to sit down in the armchair beside the door. What I did not know was that I had fallen asleep and fallen on the ground.

The following night my daughter came downstairs. She hadn't seen me all day. I usually get up on Saturday mornings to visit my sister, so it was unlikely for me to be home all day. I had come in Friday night and gone straight to bed, so by Saturday I should have been out and about.

My daughter usually comes to see me so we can catch up on the week, and I would tell her about her aunt. When I heard her scream, "Mommy!" I lifted my head and looked at her. I knew she had run from the room to call 9-1-1. Then, I heard her telling someone to cover my feet. My feet were very important because they played a major part in my survival. In my spirit, I could hear somebody saying, "You are telling me to cover her feet at this time, as if that's important." Again, my daughter said, "Cover her feet."

I do not know how long I was with those folks, but I know I was outside in darkness. It was pitch black, blacker than a hundred midnights. I saw one of my ancestors at my head. She was holding my head like a baby and positioning my head in the head-tilt, chin-lift maneuver, but she was not giving me cardiopulmonary resuscitation. She was opening my airways. Then I saw a light, the only light. I will describe it as looking like a drawing of a sperm. It was moving frantically in front of my eyes, from left to right. It was working vigorously across my face, then to my feet. The woman at my head was working frantically. She had that look of determination; she wasn't giving up. I was sailing feet first into blackness, the tiny light kept dancing fearlessly to the rhythm of what was happening. Then it turned black. I was wrapped in a blanket of darkness.

The next time I woke up, I was being transferred to a bed. I heard a comforting voice saying, "We will put you by the window so we can take care of you without getting into anybody's way," then I went back to sleep.

When I woke up, two people were caring for me. I think I went back to sleep even before they were done. Another time, I was awakened by someone for an unknown reason. By the time I asked, it was almost two weeks later, and I found out I was in the Kessler Institute. I think the staff woke me up just to take care of me.

I was behaving like I knew what was happening, but I had no idea. While in the hospital, I was told I was cognitively sound. I was discharged as being "alert and oriented," but to this day, I cannot remember being in the hospital at all, no matter how I try to. I was behaving as if I knew what was going on, they told me. My daughter showed me videos of me instructing her on where things were and how to handle things. I would answer questions quite accurately. I saw a video of me telling one of my daughters how to handle my finances. All the while, I did not know what I was doing.

I heard that the doctors were contemplating brain surgery to relieve the swelling and pressure on my brain so my people, my ancestors, wanted me out of the hospital.

Two assistants transported me from the bed to the bathroom, just eight steps away, using a wheelchair. I tried telling them I could walk, but I could not even get out of my bed. In the bathroom, I realized I was wearing a diaper. I had defecated on myself. I did not have any sense of who I was or what was happening to me.

Afterwards, they got me dressed and wheeled me to therapy.

After a couple of days of rehabilitation, things started coming to me. I was in therapy, but how did I get there or why was I in therapy?

When in bed, I remembered that voice telling me I'd be taken care of by the window. I looked around, I wasn't directly under the window, but it was across from me where there was nothing to impede my ancestors from taking care of me. There were four beds in the room. I was in the fourth bed, closest to the nurse's station. They could come and go whenever they wanted and do whatever they wanted. At that moment, I was in a place where people would be caring for me. I did not remember passing out the night I was trying to reach my daughter. I could not remember what warranted me being in Kessler.

During my time at Kessler, I was transferred to a facility to do a series of tests. This was what I call my episode of post-stroke. I do not recall if I was told I had a stroke, but that did not mean a thing to me either way. I was sleeping and living from day to day.

After daily therapy twice a day, occupational and some cognitive therapy, I could recognize folks, but I could not recall where I had met them. Some were my family members, and some were the staff, colleagues and friends. We had conversations, but when they asked me if I remembered I did not recall.

I was told that during my stay at the rehabilitation center, my children and my grandchildren never left me. They would come every day, sometimes with their friends. I distinctly remember one grandchild and two daughters, but they all came. I was never alone.

When I was discharged from Kessler, I was transferred to a nursing home until I was well enough to go home. There I had therapy twice, sometimes three times a day. The first day I was admitted, I had a shower seated on the bath chair for safety. I was placed alone near the nurses' station. The word got out that I am a Director of Nursing. This was the first time I knew I had a working title, but it did not mean a thing to me.

My sister came from Jamaica, my granddaughter and my daughter would visit no matter what time of day or night. They still had to work so they would get home and cook for me, until eventually it was time for me to leave the nursing home.

Upon my discharge home, I had a nurse, a nursing assistant, an occupational therapist, speech and physical therapists, and a dietitian to perform their specific duties. The dietitian was cancelled because she was telling me things I should eat that were not aligned with me, since I am vegan.

The nursing assistant would bathe me, as I could not use my right hand and on my left hand, my fingers were deformed. I would have therapy every day, occupational and physical, which helped me a lot.

After the home therapy was complete, I had to attend therapy at Saint Barnabas Medical Center, the hospital where I was taken first. I had physical and occupational therapy three times per week and speech therapy twice per week. My occupational therapist would look at me strangely. One day, she asked me if I was spiritual. I did not know how to answer because I did not know where she was going with the conversation, plus I could not answer her the way I wanted to. Each time I saw her, she would look at me strangely. One day I realized I did not have her anymore and I missed her. She was very pleasant, and she kept me talking even though I could hardly talk.

One day I was talking to my colleagues, the ones who visited me in the rehabilitation facility, the ones who fed me when I did not even know. These colleagues were so distraught looking at me in the hospital bed. Their reactions were, "Look at her. She is a vegetable now." These were people who knew me, who knew how active I was. Their feeling of despondence was evident.

They referred to me as a "vegetable." Can you imagine how badly off I was?

Even the registered nurse who visited me cried when she found out I was her classmate and now her patient. She referred to how intelligent I was, but intelligence, smart or otherwise, doesn't have anything to do with illness.

In physical therapy, I was made aware that stroke patients cannot bend down, meaning their head cannot go below the heart. In speech therapy, I learned that the volume and pitch of my voice were drastically decreased.

I was made to attend sessions at the hospital for weeks. When I was discharged from physical therapy at the hospital, I attended therapy at the outpatient department. Therapy had become more than two-thirds of my daily life, and sleep was the next.

The hospital made arrangements for me to transfer therapy to the South where I could continue since I was going to stay with my brother for a while.

I packed to go South not knowing my brother was coming to move me down permanently, but when he came, I just went along without a fuss mainly because I was not fully aware of my will. I just did what I was told. By two o'clock in the morning, we had everything packed and were ready. As I hugged my daughter, the voice said to me, "You are not to come back up here again. You will spend six months in your brother's house." I just walked away. My heart was in my mouth because I was leaving everything I owned, my children, and all. The pain was unbearable, but no one knew.

The beginning of my stay down South was just about manageable, until things started happening, very unsettling things. I was contemplating selling my house. I was thinking of the best thing to do, if I should leave it with my daughter(s) to take care of. Then, once again, that voice came in the night. The voice said, "You sell that house." They even showed me the money I would get. The voice said, "You take it or else you will have a hard time. Moreover, you don't want to keep it. It will not be well with you if you do." I was still having trouble deciding what would happen to my daughter, when the voice said, "Your daughter will be fine. You are worried about her, but she will be alright. This will give her the chance to make a good life for herself. She may think you are abandoning her now, but she'll understand."

In the morning, I called the oldest of my daughters and told her to sell the house.

Some things did not work out. I decided to stop going to therapy at the hospital. It had gotten too complicated because I had to depend on someone to take me. I kept cool, and I prayed. It was not my intention to cause ruckus in a house that saved me from up north. At this time, I felt like my ancestors had told my brother to come get me, so I did not want to cause a rift.

During Christmas time, I wrote a letter to my brother's wife thanking her for all she had done. I could not talk to convey what I wanted to express. I do better with writing, even though it took half a day to write. The penmanship was not good, but it was the best I could do, considering the stroke. I had a left hemisphere stroke, and my language and speech were affected. I suffered from aphasia, the side of my brain where penmanship, reading, and talking do not function too well. I watched her read it. She said nothing. She just folded it and put it away.

I found a house not far from my brother. I was happy he would not have to travel far to see me.

Thanks to my ancestors.

I had seen this house before and I admired it, but it was not for sale then.

To my surprise, it went on the market in late November. Thanks to my ancestors, I bought it. The house was ready, but the lawyer was away for the holidays. The day he came back, my daughter came from New Jersey and we closed the deal. Remember, the voice said I would spend six months at my brother's house. I moved down on July 1st, and I stayed until January.

On January 7th, I was sleeping on an air mattress in my own house. Nobody had to come check my pulse to see if I was still alive, I didn't have to step over things I didn't want to step over, I didn't have to worry if I would eat, and I didn't have to vomit because I was hungry.

As part of my recovery, I went home for rest and relaxation, some good food, and herbal medicine. I spent ten months in Jamaica, during which time I checked with a medical doctor for examination of lab tests including strength, malaria, human immunodeficiency syndrome (HIV), stool test, and Rapid Plasma Reagin (RPR). These diseases, in the latent form can cause stroke or stroke-like symptoms. After weeks of tests, I was told, "I do see you getting better from the stroke. Everything on the outside indicated stroke but, on the inside, it is different".

I used to cry and I did not know why I cried. I asked the doctor, and he said he did not know. Later, I found out it was the pseudobulbar effect, which affects some stroke patients. Then there is the aphasic effect, and the mobility effect, which causes your body not to do the things you used to. Things would fall from my hand, and I did not even know it. My legs could not lift like they used to, they would shuffle. My nerves were wreaking havoc, especially my feet. It felt like things were creeping inside my feet to my knees. They were swollen all the way up to my thighs. My lower extremities were cold, and a strange hot feeling would radiate. At times, I could not stand or even touch them.

Nighttime, it would be so awful. I would scream and pray again, but the voice would tell me not to yell: "I must bear the sensation because healing was happening." It would start in both feet up to my knees, and travel to my right hip because I had a left-sided stroke. I prayed—I always prayed— and these times, God was my only true friend. I had no one else but God and my ancestors. I figured if God was busy, my ancestors would take care of me. So, I used to ask God, "God, if you are busy because people are calling on you, I will understand. Just give my ancestors the instructions and send them until you are ready. After all, you made them." Sometimes, when I sit down, I just call on God to come sit beside me and reason.

I am so friendly with God that He would smile while I am talking. Sometimes I just tell him, "God, I called just to tell You thanks. I don't want anything; I just call to thank

You and to remind You that You are the only friend I have, and I know that You are with me."

One night, while coming from the bathroom, I tried to get on the bed and—oops—I fell. This frequently happened. But that night, I just laughed and laughed. I find myself talking to God; I was just laughing while I talked with Him. I don't recall when or how I got off the floor, but that was the last time I ever fell.

My nursing, reflexology, holistic nursing, and a little bit of bush medicine and meditation came to help. Everything holistic comes into play. I thank God that I have learned these skills. My daddy always told us, "When you start something, finish it." I am glad I finished it all. Perhaps if I did not know these things, I would not have been able to help myself when I was on my own.

One occasion, I tried to call a doctor, but the receptionist was very condescending, so arrogant that I did not even go to that doctor anymore. I was having problems speaking, then the voice said, "Why not tell them you had a stroke?" Then I started to say, "Please be patient with me, I had a stroke." Sometimes it would take seconds, maybe minutes, for the word "stroke" to come out. I would cry because I knew what I wanted to say, but it would not come. It was in my brain and on the tip of my tongue, but the words just would not come out.

I learned through crying that I would be okay, for crying is the only way the eyes speak when the mouth cannot. Crying is a way to sing of strength.

I used to hear that patience is virtue, but its true sense came into play when I suffered from a stroke. I found out that patience, humbleness, and discipline go a long way.

After the stroke, I felt my body was going through shock. I never felt electrocuted, but that is how my body felt. It was shaking on the inside; it was somewhat painful. It felt like my body was off weirdly, being put together in a peculiar kind of way. It was something like paresthesia, and it was weird. I came to understand that it was the feeling of healing.

Sometimes I wish it would stop, but I told myself that it is healing taking place. Whenever this feeling started, I remembered the Jamaican proverb: "clench yuu teeth pinch yuu side and bare it", because it was God and my ancestors working with me. If I did not believe in Father God the Almighty and my ancestors, where would I be today?

I give thanks every day, even when I am walking on the street. Sometimes I laugh when I remember I'm talking to myself—I am only talking to God.

I remember when I came home from the nursing home, I used to write a lot of verses about death. I did not know I was writing about death until it was pointed out to me, "Why are you writing about death?"

Some of the things I have written:

"Give me a ride to Jordon
Tell them I am coming
Please hold that train I am talking
To my Jesus hold that train I am coming
If you get there before me
Just tell them I am coming
I am taking to my Jesus
mama and daddy
I am coming
Just let me talk with my Jesus
I am coming to Jordon"

"I will stop by Jerusalem to see
Grandfather and grandmother
Tell the train do not leave me
I will stop at Jericho to see
my aunts and uncles
And the rest of the family
Tell the train do not leave me

A STROKE OF LIFE

I am talking to my Jesus"
"Hold that train I am coming
That happy, happy train
That train we are children
Sing the redemption song
I want to be on that train
Riding that train to Jordon
Tell that train do not leave"

"I want to stop by Jerusalem
to see my grandmother
and grandfather
Then I will stop by Jericho
to see my aunt and uncles
Tell that train do not leave
I am talking to my Jesus"

(This is where I was — May 12, 2018)

From October 2017 until about the latter part of 2022, I could not recall or remember if and what we talked about.

The insight into my episode of living, dying, and living again has awakened a sense in me that every living being on the face of this earth has a time to be. Some may not have a second or third chance, but whatever you do, make this life the best.

Don't wait for tomorrow to express your love or just be with the ones you care about. BE HAPPY.

I do have some residual effects, but it's nothing compared to where I am coming from.

Again, I give thanks to my Father, the Everlasting Father God of my life. I give thanks to my ancestors and the Universe.

Thanks to my daughters and my grandchildren, who never left my side.

Thanks to Rhonda and Jackie, who fed me when I did not even know they were standing by me.

Thanks to the nurses, doctors, friends, and well-wishers. Thanks to the staff at Kessler Rehabilitation Institute, Saint Barnabas Medical Center and the staff at the Outpatient Rehabilitation Center.

Thanks to the staff at Gates Manor Nursing Home, and thanks to the visiting nurses and the rehabilitation visiting staff who guided me safely up and down the stairs in my own home during the time I did not know I would walk again on my own.

Thank you so much for helping me through my left-sided hemorrhagic stroke.

May my Father God guide you in everything you do!

RESPECT and BLESSINGS

ABOUT THE AUTHOR

I feel humbled and blessed every day of my life, to visit death's door and live to talk about it.

God is my refuge and strength.

The Universe upholds me.

My ancestors guide me.

I am a child of God; I was born *en caul*.

Not how some folks will interpret it but nevertheless— neither more nor less.

At times when the spiritual world and the physical world meet, that is when God shows His mercy

I know some people say, "I believe in God," but I am that person who tells God, "Sit beside me so we can talk." Another time, I call on Him: "God, I don't have anything to say; I just want to say thank you, thank you, and thank you." And He will smile, sit with me for a little while, then leave.

Simply, I just want you to understand I always believed in God, but working two and at times three jobs, I was not attuned, nor did I dedicate the time other than to say thank you for waking me up after my fifteen-minute nap to go to another job, or to thank Him for taking me from home to work and back, or to thank Him for blessing my children. You know, that kind of thing—before you fall asleep or before you leave the house. But today, I make the time to talk to Him or just say thanks.

I hope this simple way of illustrating what my intentions are will foster the understanding for people who have ailments or any residual effects. For those who are still adjusting to the altered lifestyle, be patient and understand that your life is yours alone, and that you must give thanks to God Almighty.

When someone seems to have an impediment, give a little time—you may be surprised to learn how much they can help you to understand.

Thank God, I was there, and I understand.

Treat others with respect—it will return to you, your children, or your children's children.

BLESSING AND MORE BLESSINGS ALWAYS!

PEACE AND RESPECT